Bibliographic information published by the German National Library:

The German National Library lists this publication in the National Bibliography;
detailed bibliographic data are available on the Internet at http://dnb.dnb.de .

Imprint:

Copyright © 2015 GRIN Verlag, Open Publishing GmbH
Print and binding: Books on Demand GmbH, Norderstedt Germany
ISBN: 978-3-668-09738-4

This book at GRIN:

http://www.grin.com/en/e-book/311022/the-affordable-care-act-a-critical-review-
of-obama-care

Murali Mg

The Affordable Care Act. A Critical Review of "Obama Care"

GRIN Publishing

Introduction

The Patient Protection and Affordable Care Act which is also referred as The Affordable Care Act was duly signed by the President of United States of America, Barack Obama on 23rd March 2010. The act allows and ensures all the legal Americans to gain access to quality and affordable health care and will also create transformation within the health care system necessary to contain costs (DPC Senate, 2010). As stated by HSS, the affordable care act would likely to put the customers' in charge of their own health which in turn provides a great degree of flexibility and stability and they can be wise informed decisions about their health concerns. The ACA act also prohibits of any denial of coverage and claims based on pre-existing conditions as well as insurance taxes and penalties for insurance carriers, businesses, and individuals (Jones, 2014).

The PPACA

Well, the act is bit complicated that comprises of 907 pages with additional 55 pages, however the essence of the law is to reform and change the pre-existing healthcare system by providing more Americans with affordable quality health insurance and eradicating the spending on the U.S. healthcare. These reforms comprises of new rights and protections, benefits and rules for the Insurance firms, taxes, tax breaks, spending, funding, education and many other reforms (Obama Care Facts). It's pretty simple, the act focuses on reforming the current U.S healthcare system and the legal citizens of America would have access to better quality and affordable health insurance by possessing new powers, benefits, rights and protection. The PPACA is comprised of 9 titles that addresses essential reforms;

1. Quality, affordable healthcare for all Americans

2. The role of public programs

3. Improving the quality and efficiency of healthcare

4. Prevention of chronic disease and improving public health

5. Health care workforce

6. Transparency and program integrity

7. Improving the access to innovative medical therapies

8. Community living assistance services and support

9. Revenue provisions. (DPC SENATE, 2010)

All of the above nine titles focuses on enhancing and improving each essential reform components that are addressed above.

Critical Review

The ACA also nicknamed as Obamacare, was enacted with the main aim of improving and reforming the healthcare sector of the United States, however, there are certain compelling arguments arguing that the ACA act didn't make its mark. As stated in the report by (Forbes, 2014), the ACA law is not failing or falling, but it has skyrocketed the premiums and the healthcare has been more costly than ever, and it would have been better without the Obamacare. However, its due to the Obamacare or the ACA act, a million jobs have been created in the healthcare industry.

Since the ACA law enactment in 2010, around 982,300 jobs have created which contradicts the argument that stated once the ACA law is a job killer (Bureau of Labor Statistics, 2014). Contradictorily, the ACA act would likely to put costs on the American citizens and is more advantageous for the insurance companies. As the law dictates that everyone should have a health insurance policy, else the penalty shall be inferred upon one who doesn't have it.

These would likely to push the citizens forcibly to buy insurance policies. The insurance companies having a large group forced customers in the market, they would likely the hike the prices of the policies to higher premiums, which hinders the very goals of the ACA law (Forbes, 2014). (Moody, 2014), the Obamacare not only threatens bottom-lines of the insurers, but also the pocketbooks of the customers'. The ACA act also urges to replace the existing healthcare policies with new policies that are in line with the minimal value requirement of an ACA law. The pre-existing policies are likely to become obsolete and this would financially impact the consumers' as they have to buy a new policy which meets the federal minimum value and affordability standards.

According to the report by (Rand, 2010), the ACA act would or might lead to the consumer financial risk situation. As the newly insured would buy new insurance policies and spend more on healthcare, they would likely to face a lower risk of very high expenditures and can utilize more services. But this is the benefit only for the newly insured groups which due to the advent of the policy change. However, the law has both positive and negative effects.

Due to the ACA reform, there is considerable amount of decrease in the uninsured and increase in the insured groups. During the ACA implementation in 2009, there were around 50.7 million uninsured individuals, whilst after the implementation there were around 30 million uninsured in 2010. Out of 27.8 million of uninsured individuals, around 6.6 million people got insured by their employers which is due to the ACA reform (Jones, 2014). The act allows the parents to add up their children's underage of 26 to the policy plans, which would create profit blocks for the insurance companies (Department of Health and Human Services). As stated by the U.S Economist (Amadeo, 2014) the ACA act would also provide tax credits for the middle-class states that are required to set up insurance exchanges, which makes easier to shop health plans.

The Affordable Care act also aims at strengthening the public health and medical sectors. According to the (The Whitehouse), the administration allocated $500 million in funds to Prevention and Public Health Fund, to support activities such as community initiatives and the development of public health infrastructure. Such a program is likely to improve the medical community, as it offers for wide developmental programs. These investments also raised the number of clinicians with a clinging high percent of 300% during 2011 when compared to 2008. Also, the initiative added 18,600 new full-time job opportunities within the medical community. During 2014, around $1.5 billion was spent to incentivize careers in primary medical care in underserved communities (PwC, 2014). The ACA act also led to the development of tele health industry services that connects patients and clinicians via technology, this outlines the impact of ACA on new business development in the medical sector.

The ACA act also has a considerable impact on the employers. According to the law, the companies employing with more than 50 fulltime employees, must insure their fulltime employees, pay a penalty, or pay an employer shared responsibility fee. Else the employer should pay a penalty of $2000 per employee. The act also impose penalty on the employers of more than 100 employees, if they don't provide coverage for their employees. The below graph shows the costs impact on employers due to ACA act.

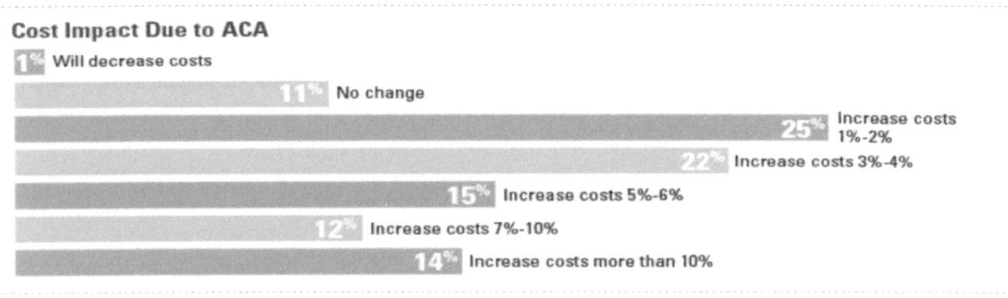

Graph 1: Adapted from IFEBP. Cost Impacts. IDEBP.2014

Small business employers have be significantly effected due to the ACA act. As stated by (National Federation of Independent Business), small employers are experiencing high costs due to offering coverages to their employees and the firms are finding it difficult to offer health coverage for their additional employees. The report from the (IFEBP, 2014) also states that more than half of the employers are not satisfied with the Affordable Care Act and the act has an negative effect on the company.

Whilst some employers trying to cope up with the situation, yet they don't know how to cope up; some number of employers are making some efforts to cope with negative effects of ACA with the below measures;

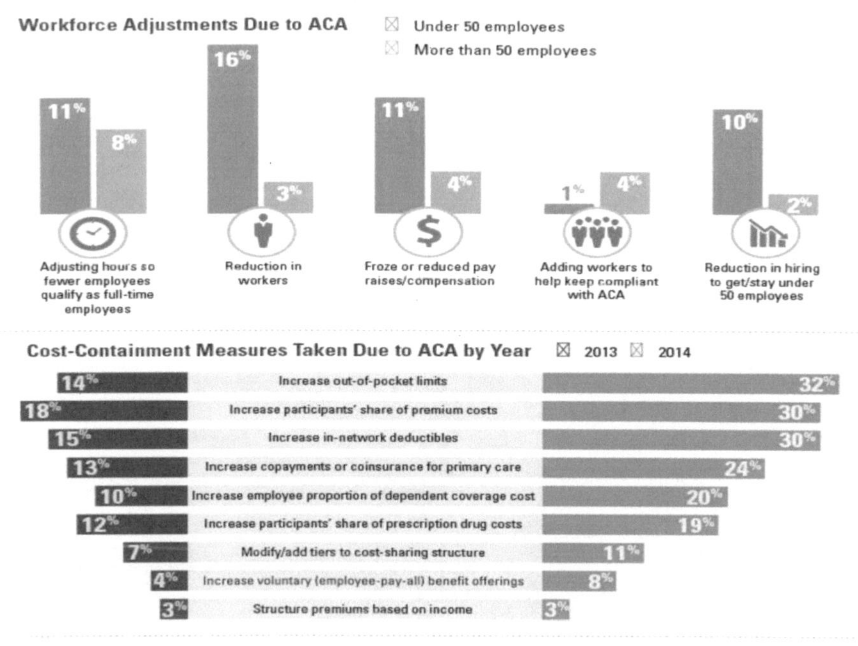

Graph 2: Adapted from IFEBP. Containment Measure. IFEBP,2014.

There is also situation that the employers will be put in a situation where they can no longer able to offer health coverages for their employees which was presented in the same report by (IFEBP,2014).

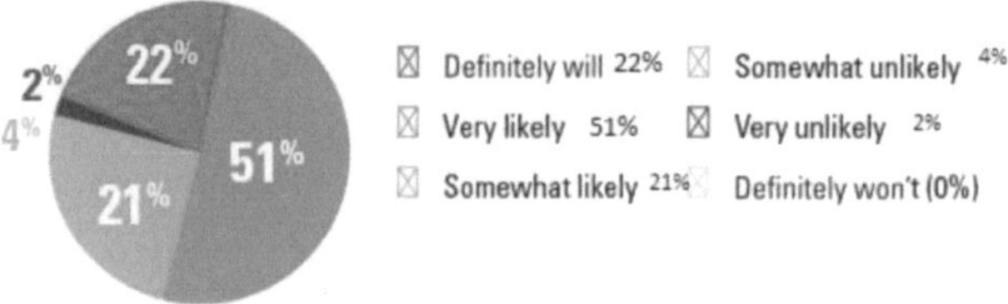

Graph 3: Adapted from IFEBP. Likelihood of Offering Coverage for Next Five years. IFEBP, 2014.

The ACA act has been argued as the "insurance company friendly" as in where the insurance companies gets the most of the flexibility in deciding the premium charges, and this is not much liked by the individuals and the citizens of America. Since 2008, the premium of the health insurance has grown over $3000, instead of reducing it to $2500 which was promised by the President (Housing Committee of Energy and Commerce).

State	Premium Increase	State	Premium Increase	State	Premium Increase
Alabama	61%	Louisiana	56%	Ohio	55% to 106%
Alaska	30% to 80%	Maine	40%	Oklahoma	65% to 100%
Arizona	65% to 100%	Maryland	34 % to 39%	Oregon	27% to 55%
Arkansas	61% to 100%	Massachusetts	39%	Pennsylvania	39%
California	42% to 61%	Michigan	35% to 65%	Rhode Island	8% to 39%
Colorado	19% to 41%	Minnesota	29% to 56%	South Carolina	61%
Connecticut	39% to 64%	Mississippi	61%	South Dakota	56%
Delaware	61%	Missouri	61% to 106%	Tennessee	61% to 100%
Florida	61%	Montana	61%	Texas	35% to 65%
Georgia	61% to 100%	Nebraska	61%	Utah	56% to 90%
Hawaii	56%	Nevada	50% to 56%	Vermont	***
Idaho	65% to 100%	New Hampshire	19% to 39%	Virginia	75% to 82%
Illinois	61%	New Jersey	39%	Washington	39%
Indiana	61% to 106%	New Mexico	56%	West Virginia	56%
Iowa	56% to 100%	New York	***	Wisconsin	34% to 106%
Kansas	61%	North Carolina	61%	Wyoming	61% to 100%
Kentucky	65% to 106%	North Dakota	56%		

Table 1:Adapted from Minsitry of Energy and Commerce. Incerease in premiums. 2013

The above table explains the premium increase during 2013. There is no decrease in premium fees, which would likely to financially impact almost all the citizens. In cities like, Chicago, Phoenix, Atlanta, and other cities, the premiums are expected to raise over by 150% on young adults which is a bad news for the buyers. The ACA act also threatens the senior citizens and these group feels that they don't get very access to the doctors, treatment options, and insurance plans as because skyrocketed premiums. According to the stats, the savings from Medicare that amount for $700 billion is saved and spent on funding new initiatives that are adhered by the ACA law, however, most of the senior citizens rely on Medicare. Such an attempt would likely to cause huge financial impact on them. Due to ACA many individuals might have to lose their company sponsored health insurance as many firms opt to pay penalties than paying for their employee's coverage.

As argued earlier, the ACA act has a considerable impact on the organizations too. If the small employers find it difficult to offer a coverage for their employees, they would likely to cut the overheads to cope up the with financial crunch situations, so that they could offer a coverage for their employees. The firms may reduce the number of working hours to below 30, so that they no need to offer coverage, which directly hits the production and indirectly influences the economic conditions of the organization. The firms might even lay off the workers, so that they don't have offer any additional coverages. As stated by (CBO, 2013), due to ACA the number of hours worked would be reduced by 2%, as the employees will have choose to work less hours which would also influence the economic situation of the company.

As the ACA act gives a wide range of access and rights for the citizens, this would create overflow of the patients to the hospitals. The increase numbers would also require more hospitals, equipment, and so on. The hospitals have invest additionally and pay taxes, as there exist 2.5% tax on purchase of medical equipment. The law also holds the payments to the hospitals for the period of 30days as a stipulation, which likely to created and economic imbalance. As argued by (Baker, 2014), due to ACA the doctors would have to see lower payments. Such situations would also result in an economic impact on the GDP, as because the American Hospitals that are around 5700 plays a major role in contributing to GDP of the nation. During 2013, medical device manufacturers paid a service tax of 10% as a training and exercise tax, which additional. This would result in the discouragement of the business doers and stops them hiring new people.

Bibliography

Amadeo, & Amadeo, K. (2015). *Is Obamacare Worth It?. About.com News & Issues*. Retrieved 28 April 2015, from http://useconomy.about.com/od/healthcarereform/a/Obamacare-Pros-And-Cons.htm

Forbes,. (2014). *Obamacare Has Failed To Collapse -- But Its Premiums Continue To Climb*. Retrieved 28 April 2015, from http://www.forbes.com/sites/theapothecary/2014/09/14/obamacare-has-failed-to-collapse-but-that-doesnt-make-it-a-success/

Harpaz, J. (2015). *Health Insurance Companies' Arranged Marriage With The IRS. Forbes*. Retrieved 27 April 2015, from http://www.forbes.com/sites/joeharpaz/2014/03/21/health-insurance-companies-arranged-marriage-with-the-irs/

House Committee on Energy and Commerce, Ministry Staff,. (2013). *The Price of Obamacare's Broken Promises*. Washington D C.

Howard, P. (2012). *The Impact of the Affordable Care Act on the Economy, Employers and Workforce*. Manhattan.

International Foundation of Employee Benefit Plans,. (2015). *Employer Sponsored Health Care: ACA's Impact*. Brookfield· IFFBP,

Jones, D. (2013). *The simple reader's guide to understanding the affordable care act (ACA) health care reform*. Bloomington, IN: Abbott Press.

Mangan, D. (2014). *Obamacare delay: Smaller employers get reprieve. CNBC*. Retrieved 29 April 2015, from http://www.cnbc.com/id/101393331

Mangan, D. (2014). *Obamacare changes a negative for insurers: Moody's. CNBC*. Retrieved 27 April 2015, from http://www.cnbc.com/id/101414902

Obamacare Facts,. (2015). *Affordable Care Act Summary*. Retrieved 27 April 2015, from http://obamacarefacts.com/affordablecareact-summary/

PwC,. (2015). *HealthCare reform: Five trends to watch as the Affordable Care Act turns Five*. PwC.

Rand Org,. (2010). *Analysis of Patient Protection and Affordable Care Act (H.R. 3590)*. California: Rand.

The Economist,. (2013). *Prescription for change*. Retrieved 30 April 2015, from http://www.economist.com/news/business/21580181-americas-hospital-industry-prepares-upheaval-prescription-change

The Patient Protection and Affordable Act. Retrieved 28 April 2015, from http://www.dpc.senate.gov/healthreformbill/healthbill04.pdf

YOUR KNOWLEDGE HAS VALUE

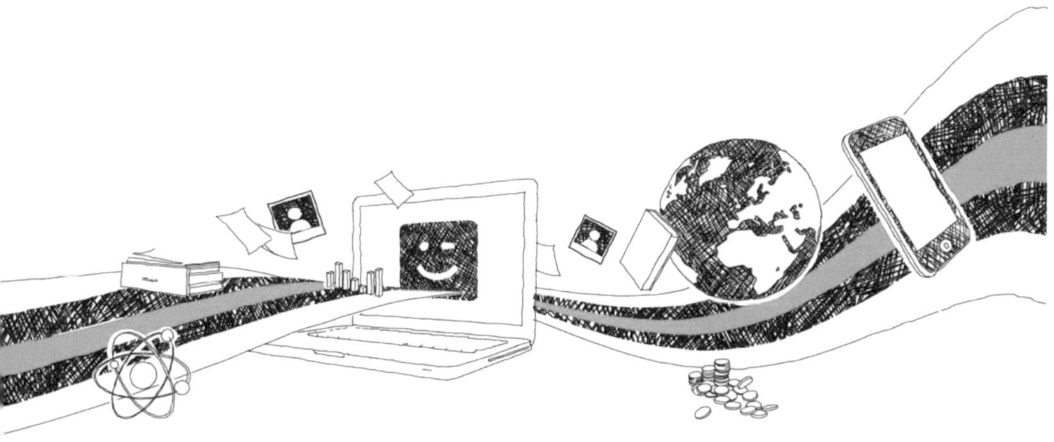

- We will publish your bachelor's and
  master's thesis, essays and papers

- Your own eBook and book -
  sold worldwide in all relevant shops

- Earn money with each sale

Upload your text at www.GRIN.com
and publish for free

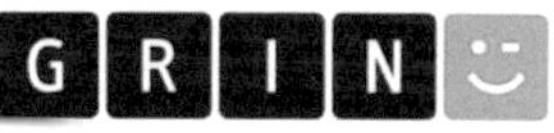